My Daily Food and Fitness Pal Journal

**MY DAILY LOG FOOD & FITNESS
PAL JOURNAL**

ISBN: 978-1-7379058-0-6 (HARDCOVER)
978-1-7379058-1-3 (Paperback)
978-1-7379058-2-0 (EBOOK)

Front cover and interior image by Dilcia Granville, Ph.D.
Dr. Granville has a background on Public Health, health, manage nutrition, that spans for over three decades. She was an Investigator/Inspector, and Public Affairs Specialist/Spokesperson with the U.S. Food and Drug Administration (FDA)

First printing edition 2021.

www.dilciagranvilleconsulting.com
dilgranville@dipandsee.com

Book about goals planner to achieve goals, there are several scheduled agendas, tips and guidances, reflections, and can be filled in as you wish

Book about goals planner to achieve goals, there are several schedule agendas, tips guidances, and reflections, and can be filled in as you wish

My Daily Food and Fitness Pal Journal

Name:______________

Date:______________

Book about goals planner to achieve goals, there are several schedule agendas, tips guidances, and reflections, and can be filled in as you wish

My Daily Food and Fitness Pal Journal

Date: .... Month: .... Year: ....

Self-Care list

....

....

....

....

Priorities:

....

....

....

....

Dear Self: ....

....

....

Things that made Me Happy Today:

....

....

....

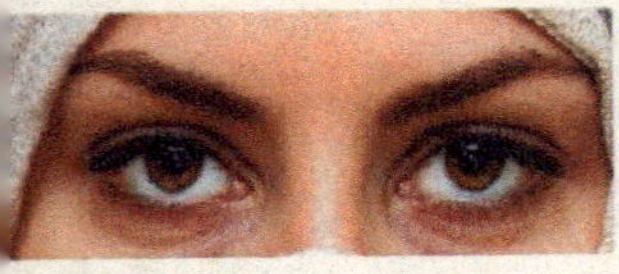

"The Greatest Wealth is Health." Vigil

CHECK-UP LISTS FOR OVERALL HEALTH AND WELLBEING

Like eating nutrient-rich foods, exercising regularly, and getting the quality anc quantity of sleep you need—all of which can boost our immunity while helping us feel our very best.

And this is exactly what we all want.

Because we understand that good health fuels your day, gives vitality to your years and most importantly, empowers you to live the life you want. Schedule appointments with your health care providers, PRONTO! That way you can make the most of your health.

- While routine, annual medical exams may be an inconvenience, they are **an important diagnostic tool that enables your doctor to keep track of any changes taking place in your body that may be indicative to an underlying disease or condition.**
- Annual exams typically check the following things, regardless of your gender:
- Medical history. Your doctor will ask you questions about your lifestyle anc habits, including smoking and drinking._______________
- Vital signs ________
- Heart and lung exams__________
- Head, neck, and abdominal exams__________
- Neurological exam___________
- Skin exam____________
- Laboratory work.____________

  Check your blood sugar, A1c________
  Check for Cholesterol___________
  Other tests____________

- Dental exam____________
- Hearing_____________
- Eyes________________

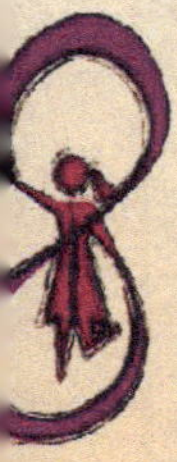

- **Women have another set of reproductive health exams that are part of annua preventative exams.**
- **Brest exam**_________
- **Mammogram**______
- **Pelvic**____________
- **Pap and HPV tests**_________

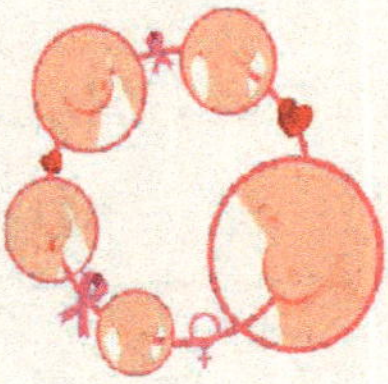

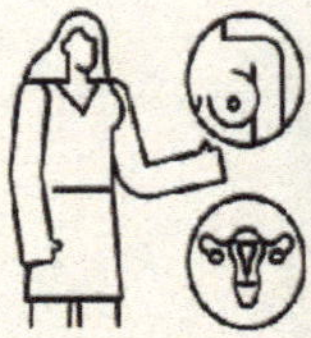

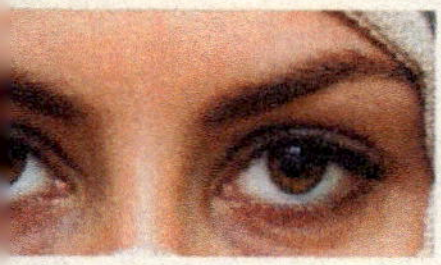

Allergies

Allergy Overview

Allergies are one of the most common chronic diseases. A chronic disease lasts a long time or occurs often. An allergy occurs when the body's immune system sees a substance as harmful and overreacts to it. The substances that cause allergic reactions are allergens. When someone has allergies, their immune system makes an antibody called immunoglobulin E (IgE). These antibodies respond to allergens. The symptoms that result are an allergic reaction.

The Asthma and Allergy Foundation of America (AAFA) has a lot of information on their website to help you learn more about allergies. Also consider, joining a local support group or contacting a regional chapter if one is in your area.

What Are the Types of Allergens?

- Drug (medicine)
- Food
- Insects that sting (bee, wasp, fire ant); bite (mosquito, tick); or are household pests (cockroach and dust mite)
- Latex
- Mold
- Pet (dog or cat urine, saliva and dander)
- Pollen

Your physician can order a blood test to find what's causing your symptoms. More often, your doctor will recommend an elimination diet, in which you stop eating one or more potential problem foods for several weeks and gradually reintroduce them one at a time.

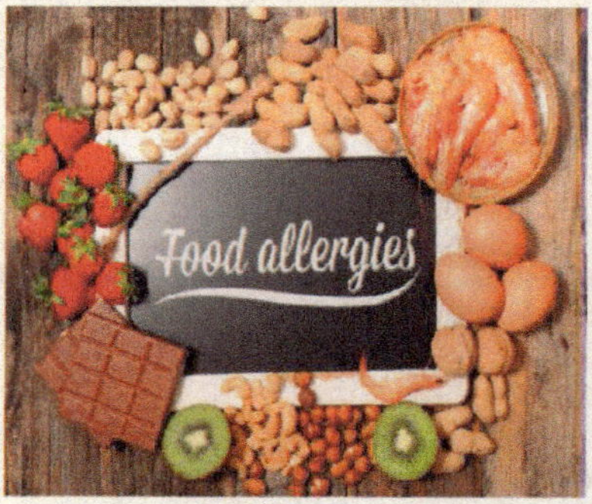

There are times when a patient thinks they are reacting to a food or having symptoms as a result of eating certain foods. In these cases, food diaries – or, perhaps more accurately, symptom diaries – can be useful diagnostic aids. These simple records of what you eat and what symptoms you feel can help your doctor narrow down possible triggers, and in turn help you feel better.

Food diaries are never used when a food is a suspected trigger of anaphylaxis (a severe, life-threatening allergic reaction) or if there is an obvious relationship between food ingestion and symptoms.

It may take a little detective work to figure out which foods trigger your allergy symptoms. But one thing that can help is to keep a symptom diaries. we have one for you, right here!

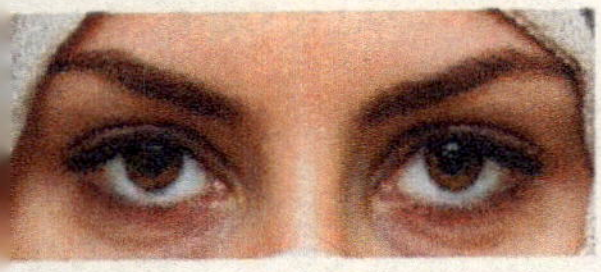

Photo Time!
Let's see that starting Photo
Date:________

My Name is ____________________

And Today I'm feeling_________________

How you look and Feel
- Speak louder about your progress -

MEASUREMENT TRACKER

S M T W T F S

Date:

Neck:

Chest:

Arm:

Waist:

Hips:

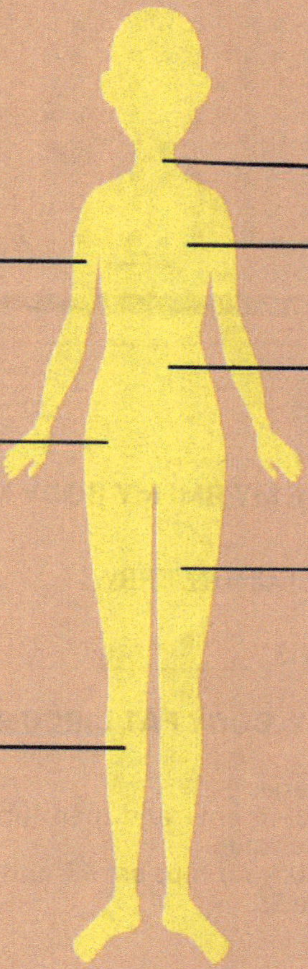

Thigh:

Calf:

Weight:

/Lbs

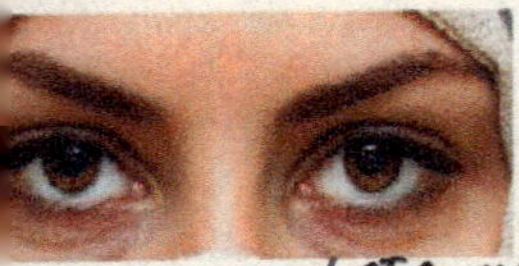

Before I start

Let's get some helpful information to help me succeed

CHECK MY BODY MASS INDEX (BMI)

HEIGHT \ WEIGHT	95	100	105	110	115	120	125	130	135	140	145	150	155	160	165	170	175	180	185	190	195	200	205	210	215	220	225	230	235	240	245
5'0"	19	20	21	21	22	23	24	25	26	27	28	29	30	31	32	33	34	35	36	37	38	39	40	41	42	43	44	45	46	47	48
5'1"	18	19	20	21	22	23	24	25	26	26	27	28	29	30	31	32	33	34	35	36	37	38	39	40	41	42	43	43	44	45	46
6'2"	17	18	19	20	21	22	23	24	25	26	27	27	28	29	30	31	32	33	34	35	36	37	37	38	39	40	41	42	43	44	45
5'3"	17	18	19	19	20	21	22	23	24	25	26	27	27	28	29	30	31	32	33	34	35	35	36	37	38	39	40	41	42	43	43
5'4"	16	17	18	19	20	21	21	22	23	24	25	26	27	27	28	29	30	31	32	33	33	34	35	36	37	38	39	39	40	41	42
5'5"	16	17	17	18	19	20	21	22	22	23	24	25	26	27	27	28	29	30	31	32	32	33	34	35	36	37	37	38	39	40	41
5'6"	15	16	17	18	19	19	20	21	22	23	23	24	25	26	27	27	28	29	30	31	31	32	33	34	35	36	36	37	38	39	40
5'7"	15	16	16	17	18	19	20	20	21	22	23	23	24	25	26	27	27	28	29	30	31	31	32	33	34	34	35	36	37	38	38
5'8"	14	15	16	17	17	18	19	20	21	21	22	23	24	24	25	26	27	27	28	29	30	30	31	32	33	33	34	35	36	36	37
5'9"	14	15	16	16	17	18	18	19	20	21	21	22	23	24	24	25	26	27	27	28	29	30	30	31	32	32	33	34	35	35	36
5'10"	14	14	15	16	16	17	18	19	19	20	21	22	22	23	24	24	25	26	27	27	28	29	29	30	31	32	32	33	34	34	35
5'11"	13	14	15	15	16	17	17	18	19	20	20	21	22	22	23	24	24	25	26	26	27	28	29	29	30	31	31	32	33	33	34
6'0"	13	14	14	15	16	16	17	18	18	19	20	20	21	22	22	23	24	24	25	26	26	27	28	28	29	30	31	31	32	33	33
6'1"	13	13	14	15	15	16	16	17	18	18	19	20	20	21	22	22	23	24	24	25	26	26	27	28	28	29	30	30	31	32	32
6'2"	12	13	13	14	15	15	16	17	17	18	19	19	20	21	21	22	22	23	24	24	25	26	26	27	28	28	29	30	30	31	31
6'3"	12	12	13	14	14	15	16	18	17	17	18	19	19	20	21	21	22	22	23	24	24	25	26	26	27	27	28	29	29	30	31
6'4"	12	12	13	13	14	15	15	15	16	17	18	18	19	19	20	21	21	22	23	23	24	24	25	26	26	27	27	28	29	29	30

Under healthy weight BMI <18.5 · Healthy weight: BMI 18.5–24.9 · Overweight: BMI 25–29.9 · Obese I: BMI 30–34.9 · Obese II: BMI 35–39.9 · Obese III: BMI ≥ 40

Weight Loss Recommendations

- For people with a BMI ≥30, weight loss is recommended
- For people with a BMI between 25 and 29.9, or who have a waist circumference greater than 40" in men and 35" in women, and who have additional risk factors, weight loss is recommended
- For people with a BMI between 25 and 29.9 who have no risk factors and do not want to lose weight, prevention of further weight gain is recommended

Risk Factors

Disease conditions:

- Established CHD, other atherosclerotic disease
- Type 2 diabetes
- Sleep apnea
- Gynecological abnormalities
- Osteoarthritis
- Gallstones & their complications
- Stress incontinence

Cardiovascular risk factors:

- Cigarette smoking
- Hypertension
- High LDL cholesterol (≥160 mg/dl)
- Low HDL cholesterol: Men <40 mg/dl; Women <50 mg/dl
- Impaired fasting glucose (110–125 mg/dl)
- Family history of premature CHD
- Men ≥45 years; Women ≥55 years (or postmenopausal)

Other risk factors:

- High serum triglycerides (>150 mg/dl)
- Physical inactivity

BMI is calculated by weight in pounds multiplied by 703 and divided by height in inches squared.

CALCULATE MY BMI MY BODY MASS INDEX

Click here: → TINYURL.COM/7N7KRRW3

MY BODY MASS INDEX (BMI) IS________________

CHECK MY BODY FAT CIRCUMFERENCE

To calculate body fat percentage,
add your waist and hip measurements, and then subtract the neck measurement to determine your circumference value.
For example, if your waist is 30, your hips are 36, and your neck is 13, your circumference value would be 53.
30 + 36= 66
66-13 = 53
My body fat circumference is _____________

What is a healthy waist circumference?

For your best health, your waist should be less than 40 inches around for men, and less than 35 inches for women. If it's larger than that, you may want to talk with your doctor about what your next steps are, including losing weight. You can't spot-reduce your waist, or any other part of your body.

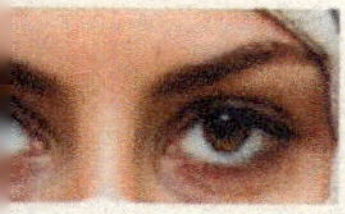

Before I start

Let's get some helpful information to help me succeed

6 ESSENTIAL NUTRIENTS MY BODY NEEDS:
CARBOHYDRATES, PROTEINS, FATS, VITAMINS, MINERALS AND WATER

In general, most adults should target their diets to comprise of
- 45-65% Carbohydrates,
- 10-35% Protein
- and 20-35% Fat.

If you're trying to lose weight, the number should be adjusted to 10-30% Carbohydrates, 40-50% Protein and 30-40% Fat.

BENEFITS OF CARBOHYDRATE

- Provides the body with fuel and energy and is found:
- Grains, fruits and vegetables, beans, dairy

Fiber-
Helps aid digestion, keep heart healthy
Found in fruits, vegetables, grains, nuts, seeds, beans

BENEFITS OF PROTEIN

- Builds and repairs muscle, organs, bones, tissues, cells.
- Helps body grow.
- Found in meat, poultry, eggs, fish, dairy products, seeds, nuts, beans, grains

BENEFITS OF VITAMINS AND MINERALS

- Vitamins are a group of substances that are needed for normal cell function, growth, and development.Different vitamins have different benefits. There are 13 essential vitamins (A, B, C, D, E, and K, with 8 vitamins in the B complex) the body requires for optimal health.
- They help heal wounds, build bones, strength immune system, repair cells and
- other functions that help our body stay healthy.
- Found in fruit, vegetables, dairy & fish
- Click for details and Recommended Daily Allowance, for vitamins and minerals

BENEFITS OF FATS & OILS

- Provide energy to our body, promote healthy cells, build strong brins, cells and tissues
- Found in butter, different types of oils

BENEFITS OF WATER

MANY REASONS WATER IS ESSENTIAL TO OUR BODIES. CLEANS THE BODY, GOOD FOR YOUR BRAIN, CELLS, DIGESTION AND OVERALL HEALTH.

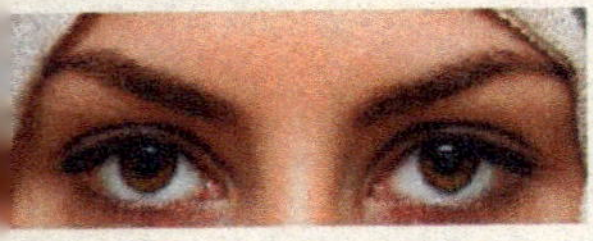

Before I start
Let's get some helpful information to help me succeed

CALORIE CALCULATOR

USE THE CALORIE CALCULATOR TO ESTIMATE THE NUMBER OF DAILY CALORIES YOUR BODY NEEDS TO MAINTAIN YOUR CURRENT WEIGHT.

click below and follow the instructions.

Mayo Clinic calorie calculator:

tinyurl.com/4pfvdn6t

My number of daily calories my body needs to maintain your current weight is__________

Lifestyle

Lifestyle changes are behavior modifications or habit changes that encourage positive changes in your life. These are a fundamental component to any wellness program. Examples of lifestyle habits include: Sleeping patterns

- Stick to a sleep schedule. Set aside no more than eight hours for sleep.
- Pay attention to what you eat and drink. Don't go to bed hungry or stuffed.
- Create a restful environment. Create a room that's ideal for sleeping.
- Limit daytime naps.
- Include physical activity in your daily routine.
- Manage worries.

Mental Health Tips

- EAT WELL FOLLOW THE PLATE
- Avoid alcohol, smoking and drugs.
- Get plenty of sunlight.
- Manage stress.
- Activity and exercise.
- Do something you enjoy.
- Connect with others and be sociable.
- Limit your screen time.

HERE ARE 8 EASY WAYS TO REDUCE YOUR SCREEN TIME:

- Eat your meals without a screen.
- Limit your non-work screen time.
- Don't watch movies or TV in bed.
- Cut down on computer socializing.
- Set a timer.
- Ban phone charging from the bedroom.
- Take up another hobby for boredom.
- Schedule a meeting phone call instead of using chat.

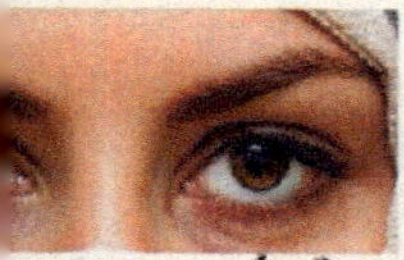

Before I start
Let's get some helpful information to help me succeed

CHECK MY PLATE
MY BODY NEEDS:
CARBOHYDRATES, PROTEIN, FAT, VITAMINS, MINERAL AND WATER

MyPlate is the current nutrition guide published by the USDA's Center for Nutrition Policy and Promotion, a graphic depicting a place setting with a plate and glass divided into five food groups. It replaced the USDA's MyPyramid guide on June 2, 2011, ending 19 years of USDA food pyramid diagrams.

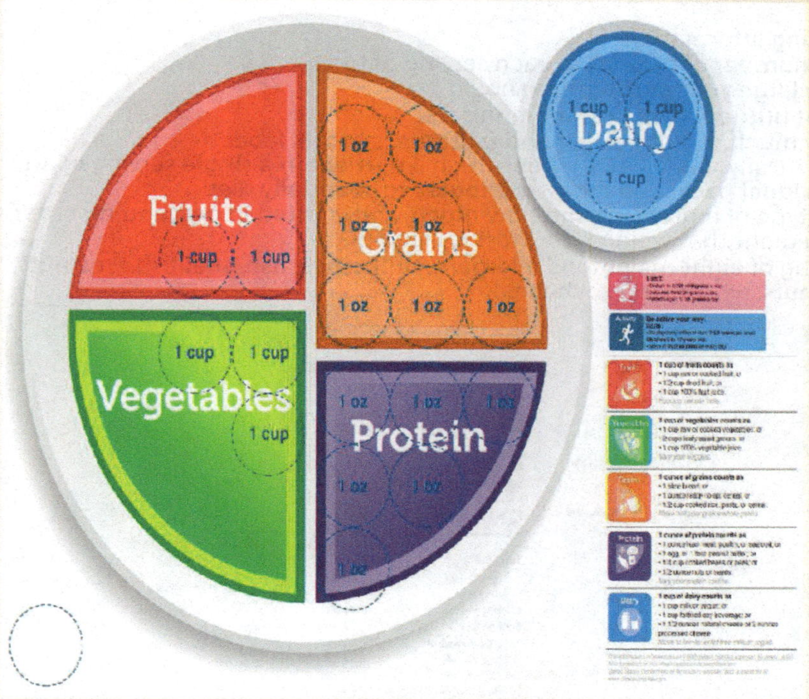

HOW MUCH CALORIES DO I NEED?

Go with an Estimate
Calorie needs for adult women range from 1,600 to 2,200 per day. For men, the estimates range from 2,000 to 3,200 per day.

Follow these guidelines to consume a nutrient-dense diet:

- Choose real food over processed food.
- Aim to cover at least half of your plate with plants (vegetables, fruit, whole grains, beans, nuts, and seeds).
- The rest of your plate should include a lean and clean protein (plant or animal) and a healthy source of fat.
- Have fun cooking at home!

Remember:
If you're trying to lose weight, the number should be adjusted to 10-30% Carbohydrates, 40-50% Protein and 30-40% Fat.

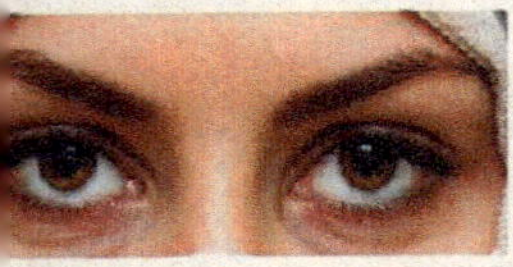

Before I start
Let's get some helpful information to help me succeed

READING THE FOOD LABEL TO KEEP IN TRACK

The recent Food Labeling by the U.S. Food and Drug Administration (FDA) updated the nation's packaging requirements to provide clear nutritional information to consumers to help make healthier and more informed purchasing decisions.

Food labels contain information like:

- Serving information
- The number of calories in each serving of food.
- How large your portion size should be.
- What nutrients are present in this item.
- How much sodium, sugar and fat there is in this food.
- The %Daily Value (%DV) -how much a nutrient in a single serving of an individual packaged food contributes to your daily diet
- The type of ingredient and how much, and is listed in descending order, the ingredient that weighs the most is listed first,
- Listing of eight major food allergens: milk, eggs, fish, shellfish, tree nuts, peanuts, wheat, and soybean.

Sample Label for Frozen Lasagna

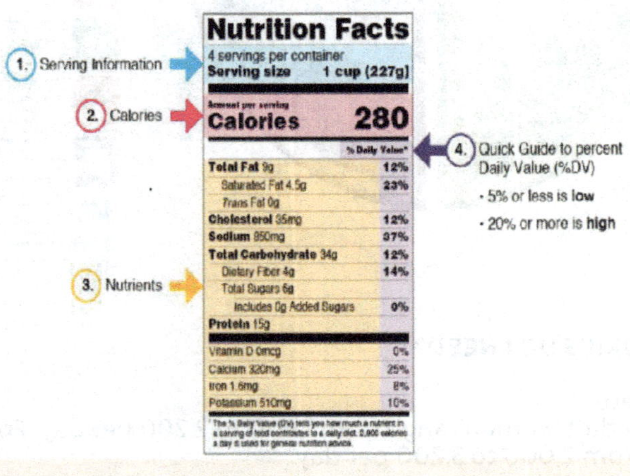

Always remember the 5/20 rule: 5% or less of bad nutrients and 20% or more of the good ones! 5% DV or less is considered low (aim low for total fat, saturated fat, trans fat, cholesterol, sugar, and sodium) and 20% DV or more is high (aim high for vitamins, minerals and fiber).

The American Heart Association (AHA) suggests an added-sugar limit of no more than 100 calories per day (about 6 teaspoons or 24 grams of sugar) for most women and no more than 150 calories per day (about 9 teaspoons or 36 grams of sugar) for most men. There's no nutritional need or benefit that comes from eating added sugar.

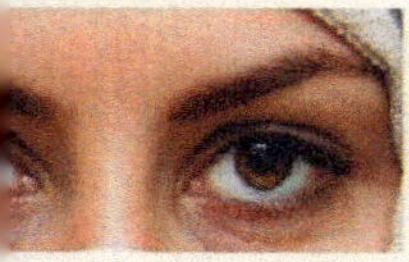

Before I start

Let's get some helpful information to help me succeed

Choosing healthy food is important

- A healthy diet is essential for good health and nutrition. It protects you against many chronic noncommunicable diseases, such as heart disease, diabetes and cancer. Eating a variety of foods and consuming less salt, sugars and saturated fats, are essential for healthy diet.

shopping Tour, Healthy & Wisely

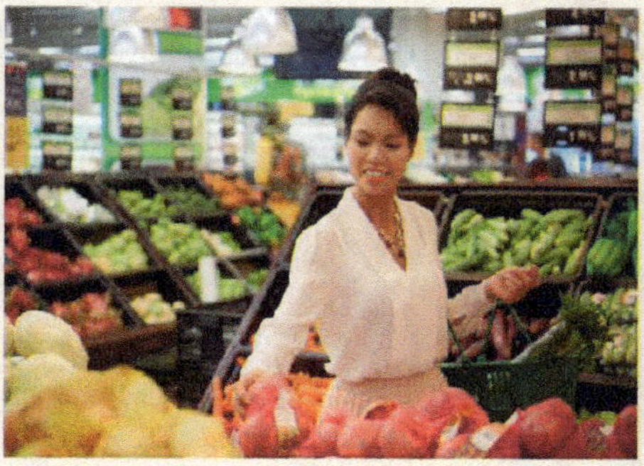

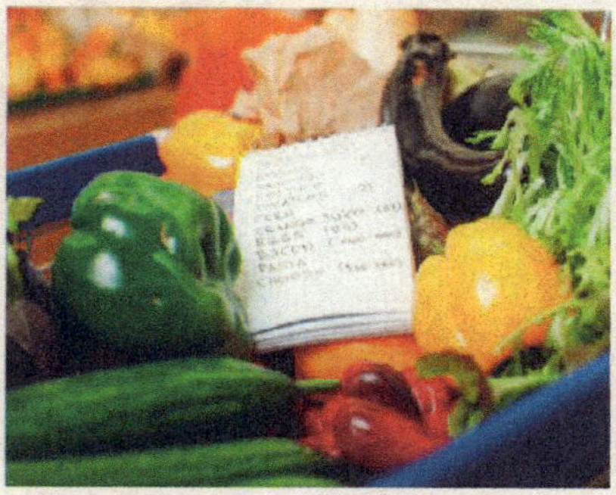

- Come prepared. Plan menus and make your list ahead of time to stay focused as you shop and avoid purchasing less-healthy items you don't need.
- Shop the outer aisles of the store first; this is where fresh foods like veggies, fruits, whole grains, dairy, fish and lean meats usually reside. Then head to the center aisles for healthy staples like frozen fruits and vegetables, canned or dry beans, and instant oatmeal.
- Spend some time exploring the produce section. Look for produce that's in season or on sale to save some money.
- Read Nutrition Facts labels, even for foods you think may be healthy..
- Don't shop on an empty stomach this can lead to impulsive purchases out of hunger.
- When buying canned fish, chicken or lean meat, look for items packaged in water instead of oil, and labeled no salt added or lower sodium.
- Buying frozen or canned fruits and veggies helps avoid food waste.
- When buying grains and bread products look for items that list a whole grain first in the ingredients instead of enriched flour or "multi-grain.".
- Divide the snacks. When you get home from the store, portion out your snack foods into individual serving sizes in snack containers or baggies.

Before I start

Let's get some helpful information to help me succeed

KEEP MOVING

Get at least 150 minutes of moderate aerobic activity or 75 minutes of vigorous aerobic activity a week, or a combination of moderate and vigorous activity. The guidelines suggest that you spread out this exercise during the course of a week. Greater amounts of exercise will provide even greater health benefit.

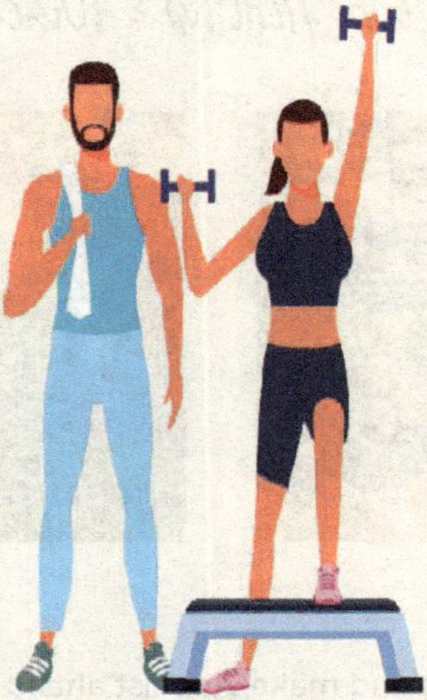

10,000 STEPS

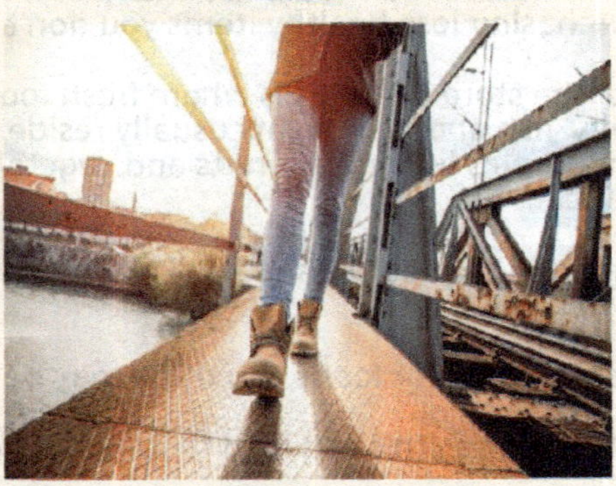

Current guidelines suggest that most adults should aim for about 10,000 steps per day . People with specific goals, such as weight loss or muscle strengthening, may benefit from increasing the intensity of walking. The benefits of walking appear to increase in line with physical activity.

Completing an extra 10,000 steps each day typically burns about 2000 to 3500 extra calories each week. One pound of body fat equals 3500 calories, so depending on your weight and workout intensity, you could lose about one pound per week simply by completing an extra 10,000 steps each day.

"Happiness is the Highest Form of Health."- Dalai Lama

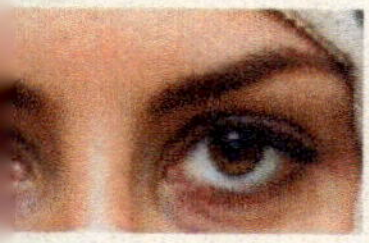

HOW TO USE MY 16 WEEKS DAILY LOG

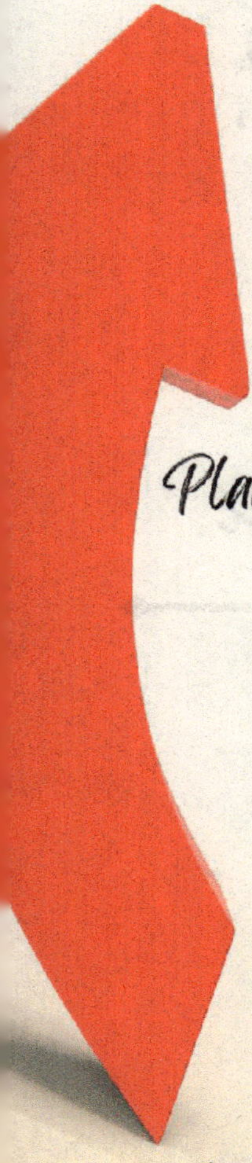

1. Define Your Goals
2. Start with your Weekly Measurement Tracker
3. Then, My Daily Fitness Planner and Steps
4. My Weekly Food Dairy Log
5. Then, Calories Intake Tracker
6. Write Personal Reflections

"The secret of health for both mind and body is not to mourn for the past, not to worry about the future, or not to anticipate troubles, but to live in the present moment wisely and earnestly."
~Buddha

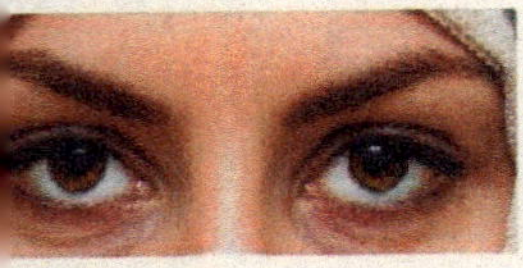

This Isn't just a term diet,

It's A

Long Term Lifestyle Chance.

Patience

Persistence

And

One Day at a Time

Define Your Goals

GOALS

ACTIONS TO TAKE

MOTIVATIONS

STEPS

POTENTIAL PROBLEMS

PROGRESS TRACKER

Motivation is what gets you started
-Habit is what keeps you going-

MY FITNESS GOALS

MY TOP FITNESS GOALS

MY MOTIVATION

	START	GOAL
Weight		
BMI		
Chest		
Waist		
Hips		
Arm		
Body Fat		
Muscle		

REMINDERS

NOTES

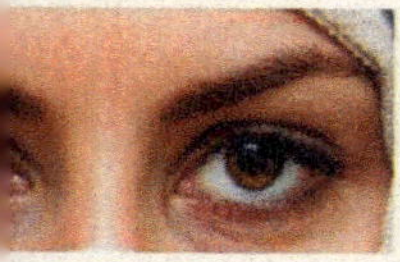

Personal Reflections

Lifestyle, Nutrition, and Fitness

Let's revisit your "WHY?"

Why are you embarking on this journey?

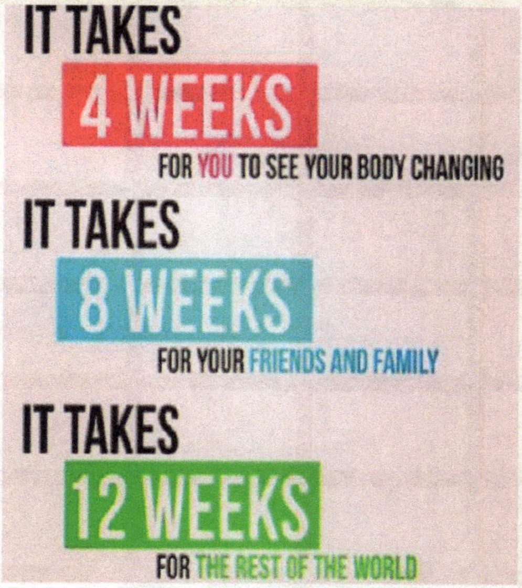

"Wisdom is doing Now what you are going to be happy with later on." -Joyce Meyer

MEASUREMENT TRACKER

My Path to Fitness

GOALS	ACTION STEPS

	WEEK 1	WEEK 2	WEEK 3	WEEK 4
Weight				
Chest				
Arm				
Waist				
Hips				
Thighs				
Calf				
BMI				

MY DAILY FITNESS PLANNER

date: ____________

GOALS

____

____

____

WORKOUTS

EXERCISE	*TIME*	*REPS*

WATER INTAKE

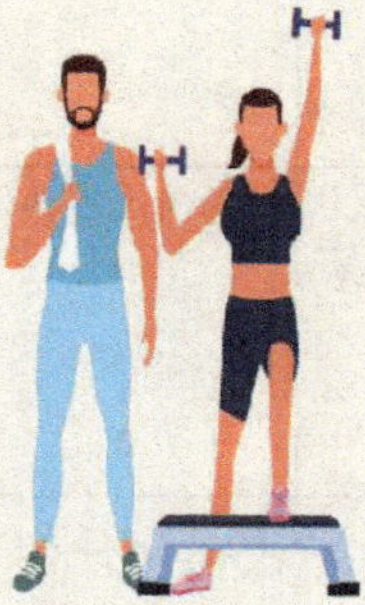

STEPS

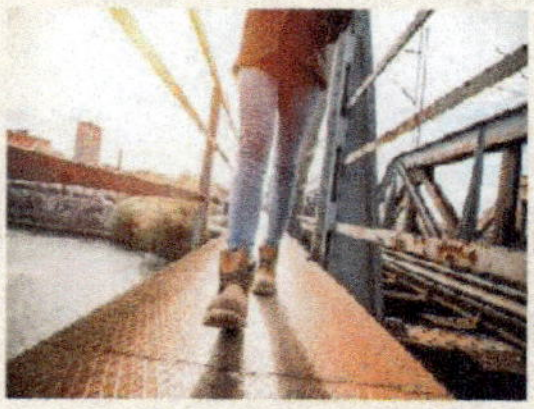

"To climb steep hills requires slow pace at first."
-William Shakespeare

My Weekly Food Diary Log
Symptom Diaries

Weekly FOOD DIARY

YEAR

____

JAN FEB MAR APR MAY JUN
JUL AUG SEP OCT NOV DEC

DATE	MEALS	SYMPTOM NOTES
MONDAY ______		
TUESDAY ______		
WEDNESDAY ______		
THURSDAY ______		
FRIDAY ______		
SATURDAY ______		
SUNDAY ______		

CALORIES INTAKE TRACKER

	Breakfast	Lunch	Dinner	Snack
SUN				
MON				
TUE				
WED				
THU				
FRI				
SAT				

Personal Reflections

Lifestyle, Nutrition, and Fitness

HABITS I NEED TO IMPROVE

THINGS I REGRET NOT DOING

HOW TO BE A BETTER VERSION OF ME

THINGS I LEARNED THIS WEEK

"If you can dream it, you can achieve it." ~ Zig Ziglar ~

MY DAILY FITNESS PLANNER

date: ____________________

GOALS

WORKOUTS		
EXERCISE	TIME	REPS

WATER INTAKE

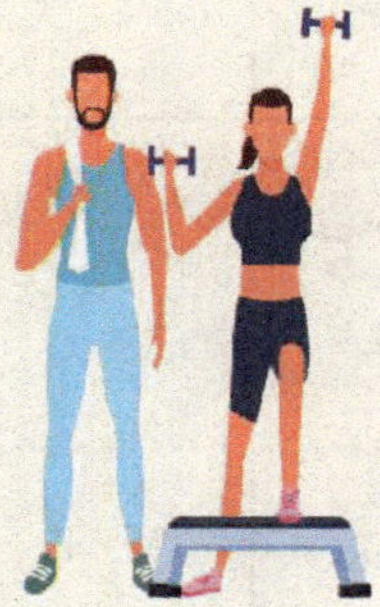

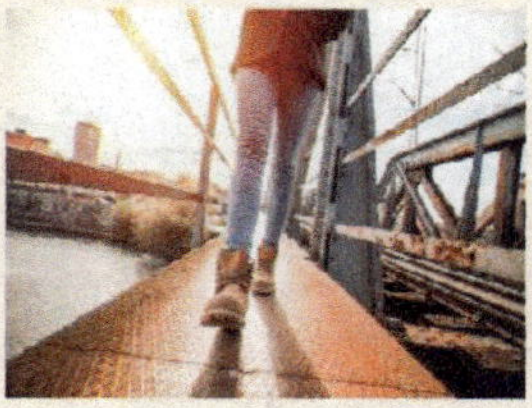

STEPS

"“Take care of your body. It's the only place you have to live.”
-Jim Rohno

My Weekly Food Dairy Log
Symptom Diaries

Weekly
FOOD DIARY

YEAR					
____________					
JAN	FEB	MAR	APR	MAY	JUN
JUL	AUG	SEP	OCT	NOV	DEC

DATE	MEALS	SYMPTOM NOTES
MONDAY _______		
TUESDAY _______		
WEDNESDAY _______		
THURSDAY _______		
FRIDAY _______		
SATURDAY _______		
SUNDAY _______		

CALORIES INTAKE TRACKER

	Breakfast	Lunch	Dinner	Snack
SUN				
MON				
TUE				
WED				
THU				
FRI				
SAT				

Personal Reflections

Lifestyle, Nutrition, and Fitness

HABITS I NEED TO IMPROVE

THINGS I REGRET NOT DOING

HOW TO BE A BETTER VERSION OF ME

THINGS I LEARNED THIS WEEK

Some people want it to happen, some wish it would happen, others make it happen.

MY DAILY FITNESS PLANNER

date: ____________

GOALS

____
____
____

WORKOUTS

EXERCISE	*TIME*	*REPS*

WATER INTAKE

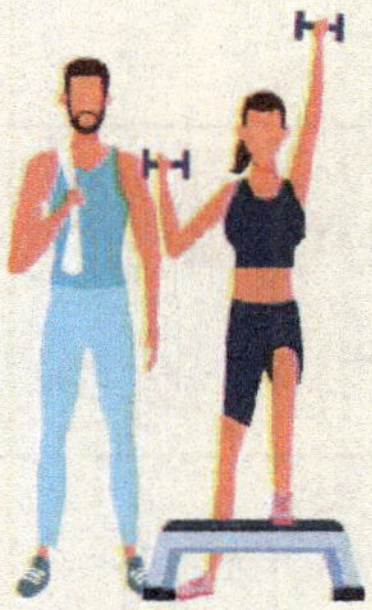

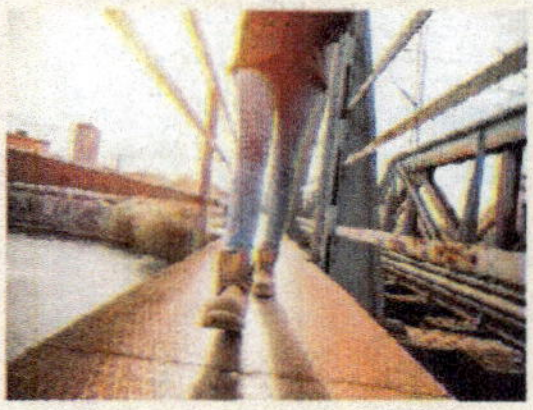

STEPS

"Self-respect is the fruit of discipline; the sense of dignity grows with the ability to say no to oneself." -Abraham J. Heschel

Food Allergies
Symptom Diaries

Weekly
FOOD DIARY

YEAR					
________					
JAN	FEB	MAR	APR	MAY	JUN
JUL	AUG	SEP	OCT	NOV	DEC

DATE	MEALS	SYMPTOM NOTES
MONDAY _______		
TUESDAY _______		
WEDNESDAY _______		
THURSDAY _______		
FRIDAY _______		
SATURDAY _______		
SUNDAY _______		

CALORIES INTAKE TRACKER

	Breakfast	Lunch	Dinner	Snack
SUN				
MON				
TUE				
WED				
THU				
FRI				
SAT				

Personal Reflections

Lifestyle, Nutrition, and Fitness

HABITS I NEED TO IMPROVE

THINGS I REGRET NOT DOING

HOW TO BE A BETTER VERSION OF ME

THINGS I LEARNED THIS WEEK

Don't Wait Until You've Reach Your Goal to Be Proud of Yourself. Be Proud of Every Step You Tale Toward Reaching that Goal

MY DAILY FITNESS PLANNER

date: ____________

GOALS

____

____

____

WORKOUTS

EXERCISE	*TIME*	*REPS*

WATER INTAKE

○ ○ ○ ○ ○ ○ ○ ○

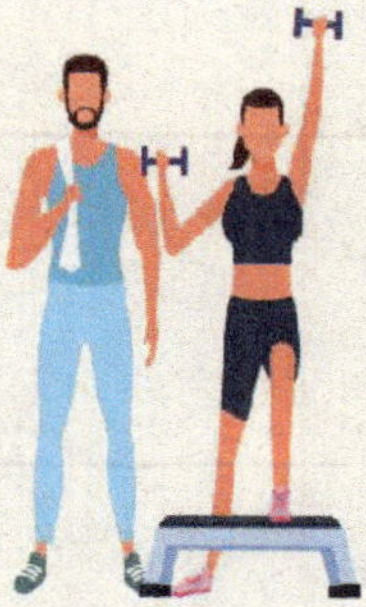

STEPS

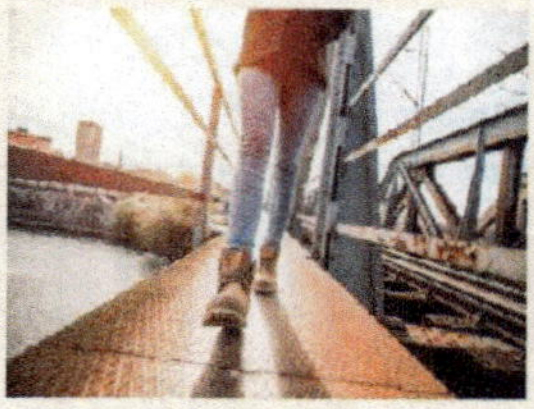

"Whatever the mind can conceive and believe, it can achieve."
-Napoleon Hil

Food Allergies
Symptom Diaries

Weekly
FOOD DIARY

YEAR					
____________					
JAN	FEB	MAR	APR	MAY	JUN
JUL	AUG	SEP	OCT	NOV	DEC

DATE	MEALS	SYMPTOM NOTES
MONDAY _______		
TUESDAY _______		
WEDNESDAY _______		
THURSDAY _______		
FRIDAY _______		
SATURDAY _______		
SUNDAY _______		

CALORIES INTAKE TRACKER

	Breakfast	Lunch	Dinner	Snack
SUN				
MON				
TUE				
WED				
THU				
FRI				
SAT				

Personal Reflections

Lifestyle, Nutrition, and Fitness

HABITS I NEED TO IMPROVE

THINGS I REGRET NOT DOING

HOW TO BE A BETTER VERSION OF ME

THINGS I LEARNED THIS WEEK

Losing weight is hard, maintaining weight is hard, staying overweight is hard. Choose your hard.

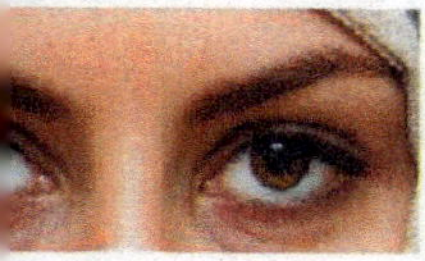

Personal Reflections

Lifestyle, Nutrition, and Fitness

Check In!

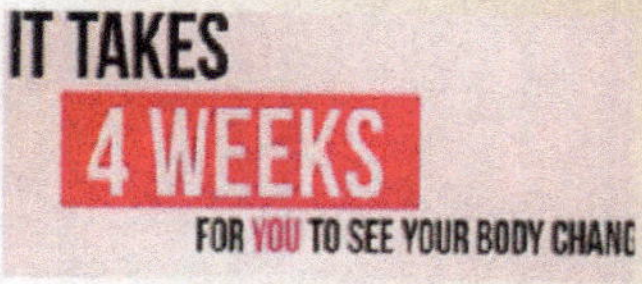

Let's revisit Why are you doing this?

Goals I have accomplished so far:

What is the One benchmark goal I hope to achieve in the following 4 weeks that will get me closer to my end goal?

Highlights the best moments of these past weeks?

What have been your biggest challenges so far?

How does it feel when you've conquered something challenging?

You must be willing to make sacrifices at times, knowing that the outcome will be worth it.

MEASUREMENT TRACKER

My Path to Fitness

GOALS	ACTION STEPS

	WEEK 5	WEEK 6	WEEK 7	WEEK 8
Weight				
Chest				
Arm				
Waist				
Hips				
Thighs				
Calf				
BMI				

MY DAILY FITNESS PLANNER

date: ______________

GOALS

WORKOUTS

EXERCISE	TIME	REPS

WATER INTAKE

○ ○ ○ ○ ○ ○ ○ ○

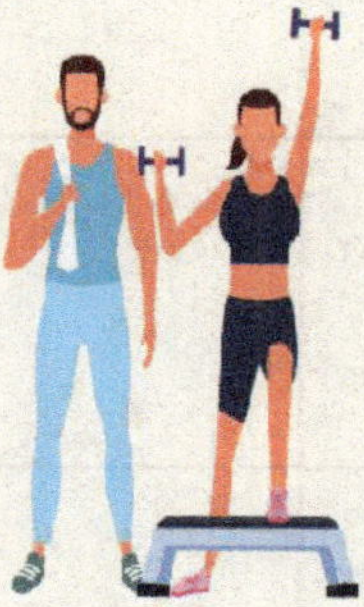

STEPS

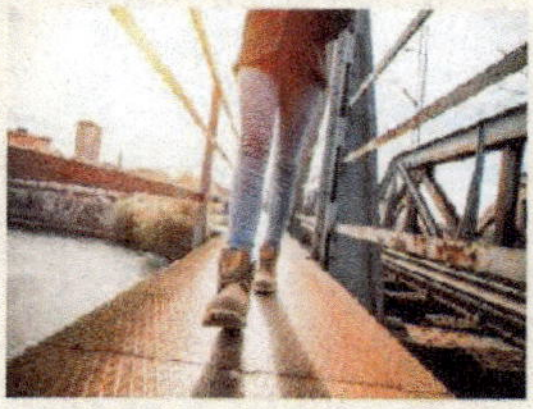

"Nothing is impossible, the word itself says 'I'm possible'!"
-Audrey Hepburn

Food Allergies
Symptom Diaries

Weekly
FOOD DIARY

YEAR					

JAN	FEB	MAR	APR	MAY	JUN
JUL	AUG	SEP	OCT	NOV	DEC

DATE	MEALS	SYMPTOM NOTES
MONDAY -------		
TUESDAY -------		
WEDNESDAY -------		
THURSDAY -------		
FRIDAY -------		
SATURDAY -------		
SUNDAY -------		

CALORIES INTAKE TRACKER

	Breakfast	Lunch	Dinner	Snack
SUN				
MON				
TUE				
WED				
THU				
FRI				
SAT				

Personal Reflections

Lifestyle, Nutrition, and Fitness

HABITS I NEED TO IMPROVE

THINGS I REGRET NOT DOING

HOW TO BE A BETTER VERSION OF ME

THINGS I LEARNED THIS WEEK

A negative thinker sees a difficulty in every opportunity. A positive thinker sees an opportunity in every difficulty.

MY DAILY FITNESS PLANNER

date: ____________

GOALS

WORKOUTS

EXERCISE	TIME	REPS

WATER INTAKE

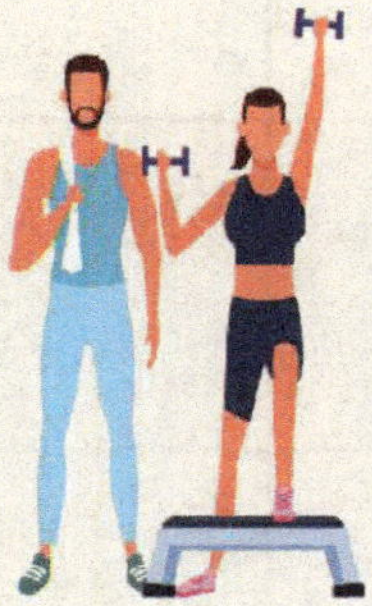

STEPS

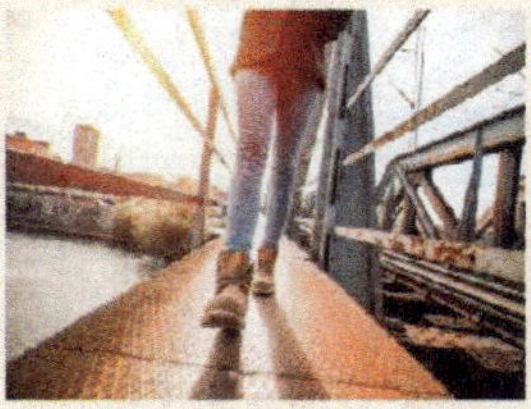

"Magic is believing in yourself, if you can do that, you can make anything happen."
-Johann Wolfgang von Goeth

Food Allergies
Symptom Diaries

Weekly
FOOD DIARY

YEAR					
___________					
JAN	FEB	MAR	APR	MAY	JUN
JUL	AUG	SEP	OCT	NOV	DEC

DATE	MEALS	SYMPTOM NOTES
MONDAY _______		
TUESDAY _______		
WEDNESDAY _______		
THURSDAY _______		
FRIDAY _______		
SATURDAY _______		
SUNDAY _______		

CALORIES INTAKE TRACKER

	Breakfast	Lunch	Dinner	Snack
SUN				
MON				
TUE				
WED				
THU				
FRI				
SAT				

Personal Reflections

Lifestyle, Nutrition, and Fitness

HABITS I NEED TO IMPROVE

THINGS I REGRET NOT DOING

HOW TO BE A BETTER VERSION OF ME

THINGS I LEARNED THIS WEEK

The older you get, the tougher it is to lose weight. Because by then your body and your fat are really good friends.

MY DAILY FITNESS PLANNER

date: ____________________

GOALS

____

____

____

WORKOUTS

EXERCISE	TIME	REPS

WATER INTAKE

○ ○ ○ ○ ○ ○ ○ ○

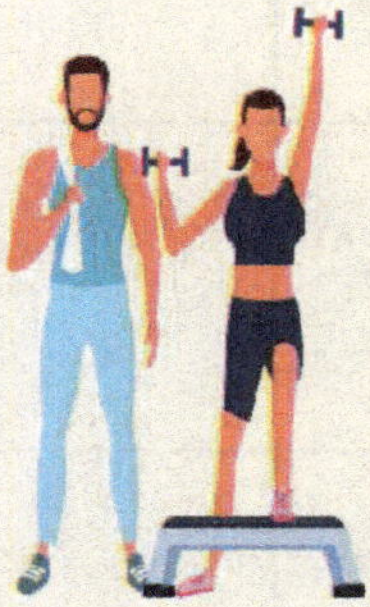

STEPS

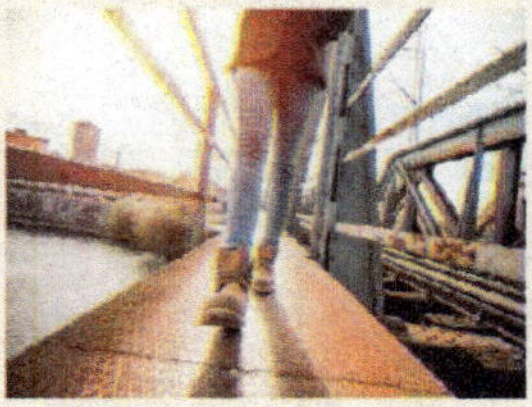

"Do what you can, with what you have, where you are."
-Theodore Roosevelt

Food Allergies
Symptom Diaries

Weekly FOOD DIARY

YEAR					
____________					
JAN	FEB	MAR	APR	MAY	JUN
JUL	AUG	SEP	OCT	NOV	DEC

DATE	MEALS	SYMPTOM NOTES
MONDAY _______		
TUESDAY _______		
WEDNESDAY _______		
THURSDAY _______		
FRIDAY _______		
SATURDAY _______		
SUNDAY _______		

CALORIES INTAKE TRACKER

	Breakfast	Lunch	Dinner	Snack
SUN				
MON				
TUE				
WED				
THU				
FRI				
SAT				

Personal Reflections

Lifestyle, Nutrition, and Fitness

HABITS I NEED TO IMPROVE

THINGS I REGRET NOT DOING

HOW TO BE A BETTER VERSION OF ME

THINGS I LEARNED THIS WEEK

Every morning you have two choices. Continue to sleep with your dreams, or wake up and chase them.

MY DAILY FITNESS PLANNER

date: ________________

GOALS

____

____

____

WORKOUTS

EXERCISE	*TIME*	*REPS*

WATER INTAKE

○ ○ ○ ○ ○ ○ ○ ○

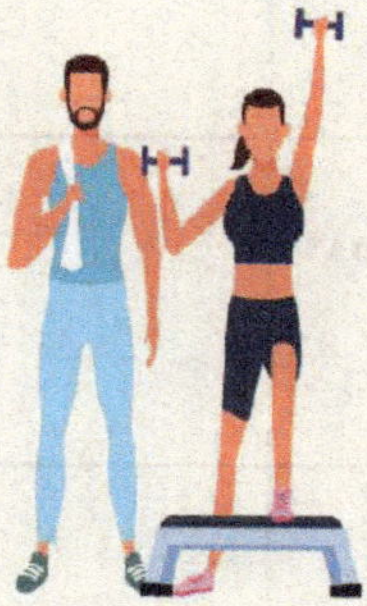

STEPS

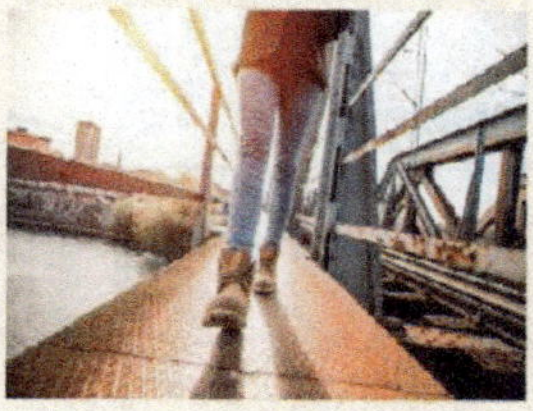

"You can't do it all yourself. Don't be afraid to rely on others to help you accomplish your goals."
-Oprah Winfrey

Weekly FOOD DIARY

YEAR					
____________					
JAN	FEB	MAR	APR	MAY	JUN
JUL	AUG	SEP	OCT	NOV	DEC

DATE	MEALS	SYMPTOM NOTES
MONDAY _______		
TUESDAY _______		
WEDNESDAY _______		
THURSDAY _______		
FRIDAY _______		
SATURDAY _______		
SUNDAY _______		

CALORIES INTAKE TRACKER

	Breakfast	Lunch	Dinner	Snack
SUN				
MON				
TUE				
WED				
THU				
FRI				
SAT				

Personal Reflections

Lifestyle, Nutrition, and Fitness

HABITS I NEED TO IMPROVE

THINGS I REGRET NOT DOING

HOW TO BE A BETTER VERSION OF ME

THINGS I LEARNED THIS WEEK

Every morning you have two choices. Continue to sleep with your dreams, or wake up and chase them.

MY DAILY FITNESS PLANNER

date: ______________

GOALS

____

____

____

WORKOUTS

EXERCISE	*TIME*	*REPS*

WATER INTAKE

○ ○ ○ ○ ○ ○ ○ ○

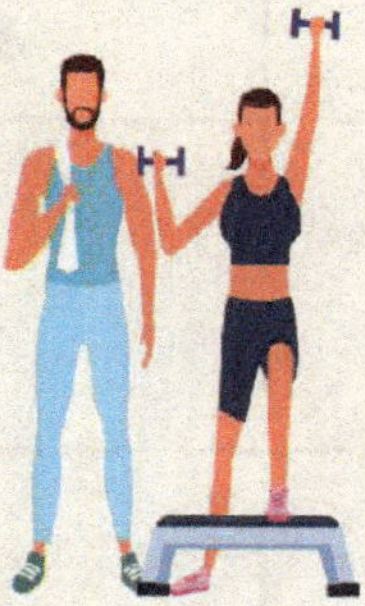

STEPS

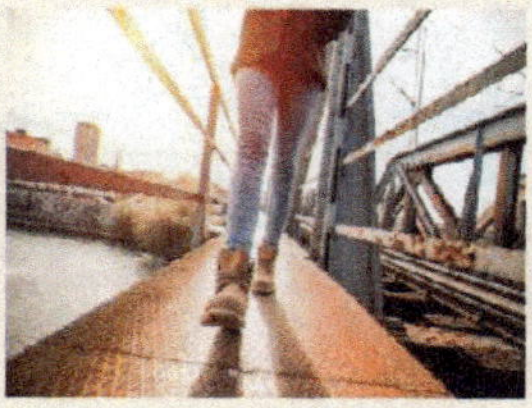

"A strong positive attitude will create more miracles than any wonder drug."
-Patricia Neal

Food Allergies
Symptom Diaries

Weekly FOOD DIARY

YEAR					
___________					
JAN	FEB	MAR	APR	MAY	JUN
JUL	AUG	SEP	OCT	NOV	DEC

DATE	MEALS	SYMPTOM NOTES
MONDAY _______		
TUESDAY _______		
WEDNESDAY _______		
THURSDAY _______		
FRIDAY _______		
SATURDAY _______		
SUNDAY _______		

CALORIES INTAKE TRACKER

	Breakfast	Lunch	Dinner	Snack
SUN				
MON				
TUE				
WED				
THU				
FRI				
SAT				

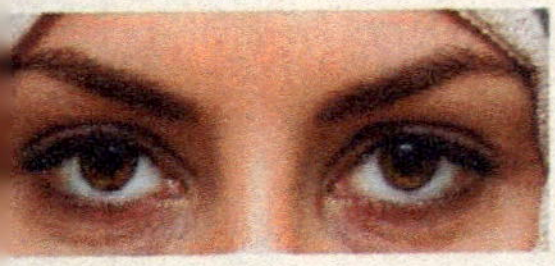

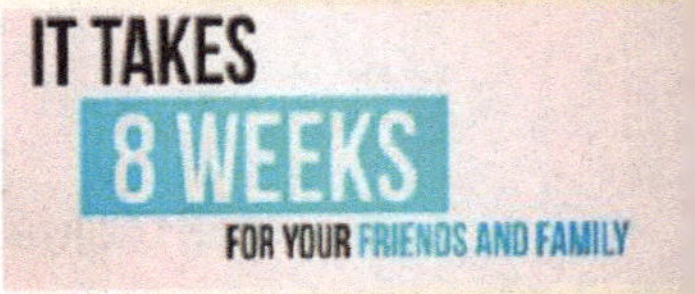

Check In!

Winners are not people who never fail, but people who never quit!

Goals Ive accomplished so far:

Highlights and/or best moments these past weeks?

One benchmark goal I hope to achieve in the following 4 weeks that will get me just a little closer to my end goal is...

What have been your biggest challenges so far?

How does it when you've conquered something challenging?

MEASUREMENT TRACKER

My Path to Fitness

GOALS	ACTION STEPS

	WEEK 9	WEEK 10	WEEK 11	WEEK 12
Weight				
Chest				
Arm				
Waist				
Hips				
Thighs				
Calf				
BMI				

MY DAILY FITNESS PLANNER

date: ______________

GOALS

WORKOUTS		
EXERCISE	*TIME*	*REPS*

WATER INTAKE

○ ○ ○ ○ ○ ○ ○ ○

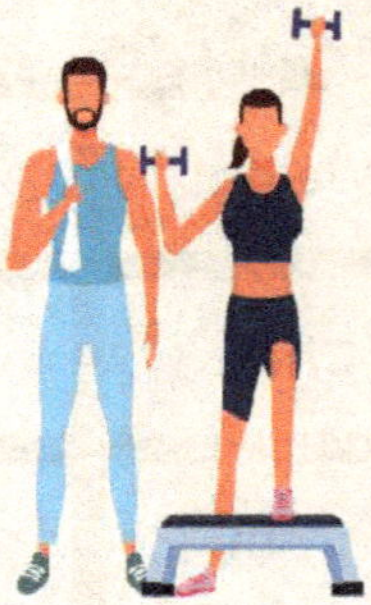

STEPS

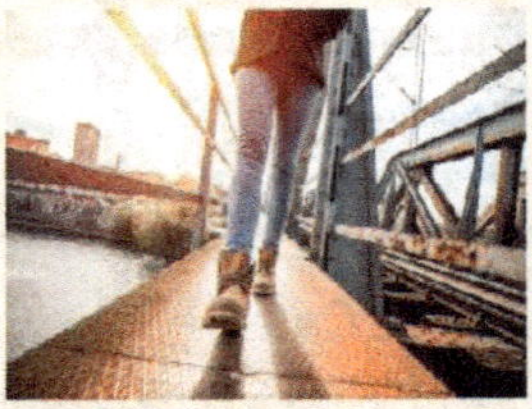

"If you change the way you look at things, the things you look at change."
-Wayne Dyer

Food Allergies
Symptom Diaries

Weekly
FOOD DIARY

YEAR

____

JAN FEB MAR APR MAY JUN
JUL AUG SEP OCT NOV DEC

DATE	MEALS	SYMPTOM NOTES
MONDAY _______		
TUESDAY _______		
WEDNESDAY _______		
THURSDAY _______		
FRIDAY _______		
SATURDAY _______		
SUNDAY _______		

CALORIES INTAKE TRACKER

	Breakfast	Lunch	Dinner	Snack
SUN				
MON				
TUE				
WED				
THU				
FRI				
SAT				

Personal Reflections

Lifestyle, Nutrition, and Fitness

HABITS I NEED TO IMPROVE

THINGS I REGRET NOT DOING

HOW TO BE A BETTER VERSION OF ME

THINGS I LEARNED THIS WEEK

It does not matter how slowly you go, as long as you do not stop.
Results come over time, not overnight.

MY DAILY FITNESS PLANNER

date: ____________________

GOALS

WORKOUTS		
EXERCISE	*TIME*	*REPS*

WATER INTAKE

○ ○ ○ ○ ○ ○ ○ ○

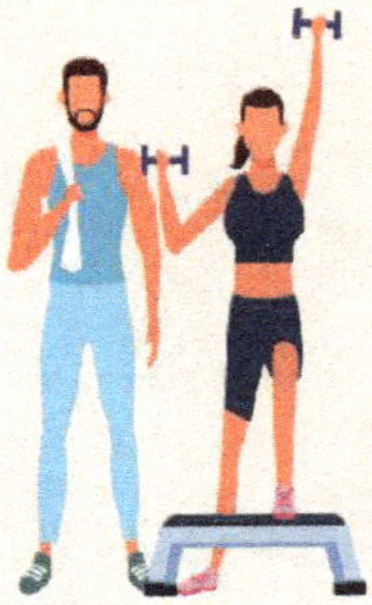

STEPS

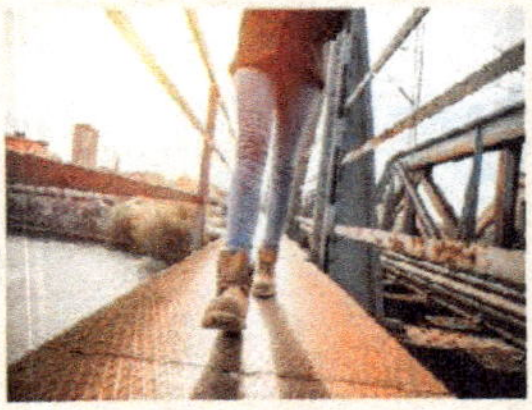

"Love yourself first and everything else falls into line."
-Lucille Ball

Weekly FOOD DIARY

YEAR

____

JAN FEB MAR APR MAY JUN
JUL AUG SEP OCT NOV DEC

DATE	MEALS	SYMPTOM NOTES
MONDAY _______		
TUESDAY _______		
WEDNESDAY _______		
THURSDAY _______		
FRIDAY _______		
SATURDAY _______		
SUNDAY _______		

CALORIES INTAKE TRACKER

	Breakfast	Lunch	Dinner	Snack
SUN				
MON				
TUE				
WED				
THU				
FRI				
SAT				

Personal Reflections

Lifestyle, Nutrition, and Fitness

HABITS I NEED TO IMPROVE

THINGS I REGRET NOT DOING

HOW TO BE A BETTER VERSION OF ME

THINGS I LEARNED THIS WEEK

I'm not there yet, but I'm closer than I was yesterday.

MY DAILY FITNESS PLANNER

date: ______________

GOALS

WORKOUTS

EXERCISE	*TIME*	*REPS*

WATER INTAKE

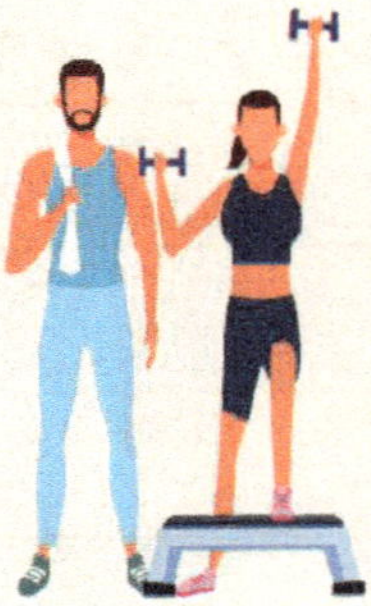

STEPS

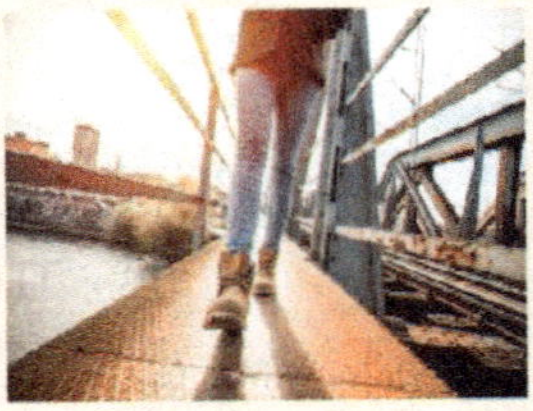

"To lose patience is to lose the battle."
-Gandhi

Weekly FOOD DIARY

YEAR

____

JAN FEB MAR APR MAY JUN

JUL AUG SEP OCT NOV DEC

DATE	MEALS	SYMPTOM NOTES
MONDAY _______		
TUESDAY _______		
WEDNESDAY _______		
THURSDAY _______		
FRIDAY _______		
SATURDAY _______		
SUNDAY _______		

CALORIES INTAKE TRACKER

	Breakfast	Lunch	Dinner	Snack
SUN				
MON				
TUE				
WED				
THU				
FRI				
SAT				

Personal Reflections

Lifestyle, Nutrition, and Fitness

HABITS I NEED TO IMPROVE

THINGS I REGRET NOT DOING

HOW TO BE A BETTER VERSION OF ME

THINGS I LEARNED THIS WEEK

I'm not there yet, but I'm closer than I was yesterday.

"Character is doing what you don't want to do but know you should do."
- Joyce Meyer

MY DAILY FITNESS PLANNER

date: ____________________

GOALS

____

____

____

WORKOUTS

EXERCISE	*TIME*	*REPS*

WATER INTAKE

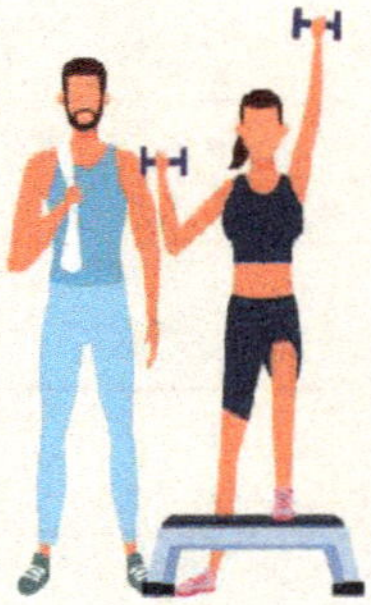

STEPS

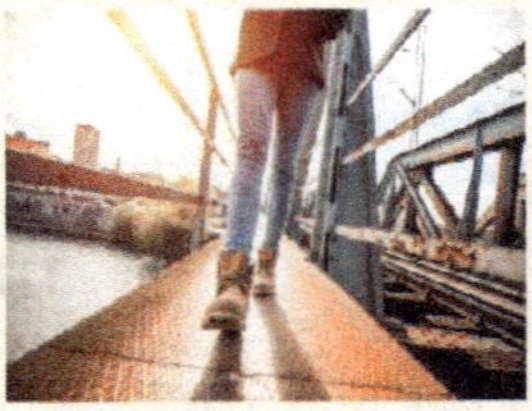

Fitness is like a marriage: you can't cheat on it and expect it to work.

Weekly
FOOD DIARY

YEAR					
___________					
JAN	FEB	MAR	APR	MAY	JUN
JUL	AUG	SEP	OCT	NOV	DEC

DATE	MEALS	SYMPTOM NOTES
MONDAY _______		
TUESDAY _______		
WEDNESDAY _______		
THURSDAY _______		
FRIDAY _______		
SATURDAY _______		
SUNDAY _______		

CALORIES INTAKE TRACKER

	Breakfast	Lunch	Dinner	Snack
SUN				
MON				
TUE				
WED				
THU				
FRI				
SAT				

Daily/Weekly Accomplishments
Reflection Time!
What went well, and What could be better
Lifestyle, Nutrition, and Fitness

"Character is doing what you don't want to do but know you should do." - Joyce Meyer

MY DAILY FITNESS PLANNER

date: ____________

GOALS

____

____

____

WORKOUTS

EXERCISE	*TIME*	*REPS*

WATER INTAKE

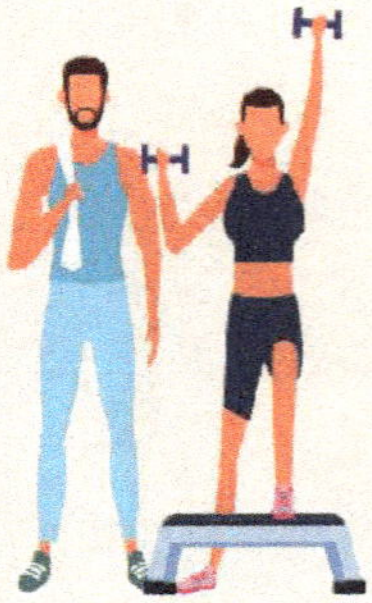

STEPS

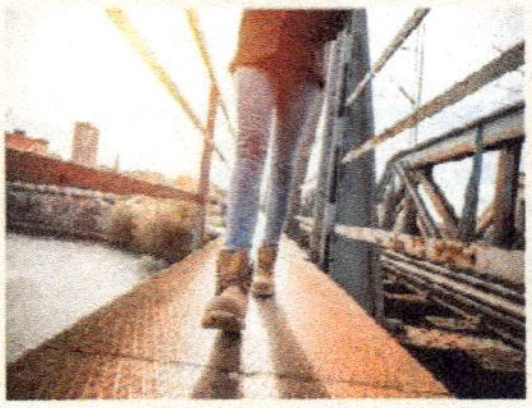

Fitness is like a marriage: you can't cheat on it and expect it to work.

Weekly FOOD DIARY

YEAR

____

JAN FEB MAR APR MAY JUN
JUL AUG SEP OCT NOV DEC

DATE	MEALS	SYMPTOM NOTES
MONDAY ______		
TUESDAY ______		
WEDNESDAY ______		
THURSDAY ______		
FRIDAY ______		
SATURDAY ______		
SUNDAY ______		

CALORIES INTAKE TRACKER

	Breakfast	Lunch	Dinner	Snack
SUN				
MON				
TUE				
WED				
THU				
FRI				
SAT				

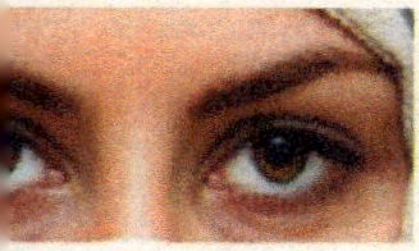

Personal Reflections

Lifestyle, Nutrition, and Fitness

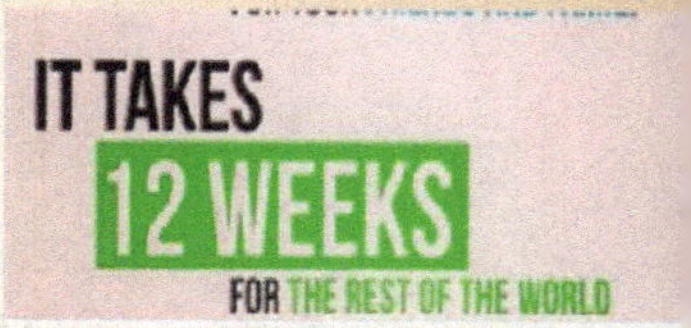

Check In!

My hard work is really starting to show!

Goals I've accomplished so far.

Higlights of the best moments these past weeks?

What have been your biggest challenges so far?

One benchmark goal I hope to achieve in the following 4 week that will bring me closer to my end goal is...?

Remember where you were when you started?

MEASUREMENT TRACKER

My Path to Fitness

GOALS	ACTION STEPS

	WEEK 13	WEEK 14	WEEK 15	WEEK1 16
Weight				
Chest				
Arm				
Waist				
Hips				
Thighs				
Calf				
BMI				

MY DAILY FITNESS PLANNER

date: ____________________

GOALS

WORKOUTS

EXERCISE	TIME	REPS

WATER INTAKE

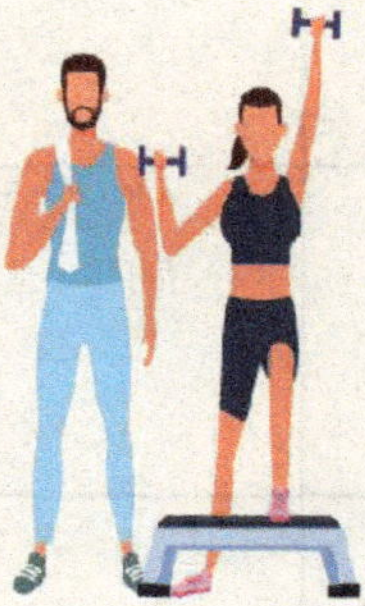

STEPS

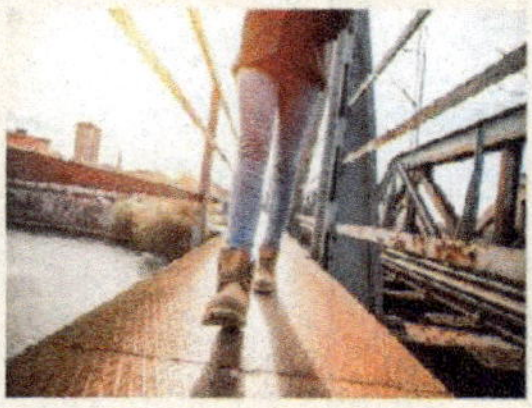

You've got the momentum, darling!
Keep up that great work!

Weekly
FOOD DIARY

YEAR					
___________					
JAN	FEB	MAR	APR	MAY	JUN
JUL	AUG	SEP	OCT	NOV	DEC

DATE	MEALS	SYMPTOM NOTES
MONDAY _______		
TUESDAY _______		
WEDNESDAY _______		
THURSDAY _______		
FRIDAY _______		
SATURDAY _______		
SUNDAY _______		

CALORIES INTAKE TRACKER

	Breakfast	Lunch	Dinner	Snack
SUN				
MON				
TUE				
WED				
THU				
FRI				
SAT				

Daily/Weekly Accomplishments
Reflection Time!
What went well, and What could be better

Lifestyle, Nutrition, and Fitness

"Free your heart from hatred. Free your mind from worries. Live simply. Give more. Expec less." ~Unknown

MY DAILY FITNESS PLANNER

date: ______________

GOALS

____

____

____

WORKOUTS

EXERCISE	*TIME*	*REPS*

WATER INTAKE

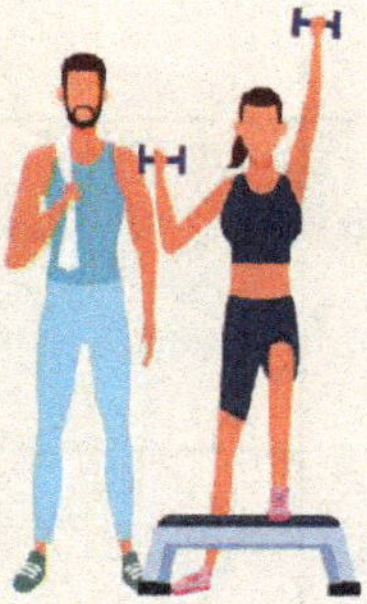

STEPS

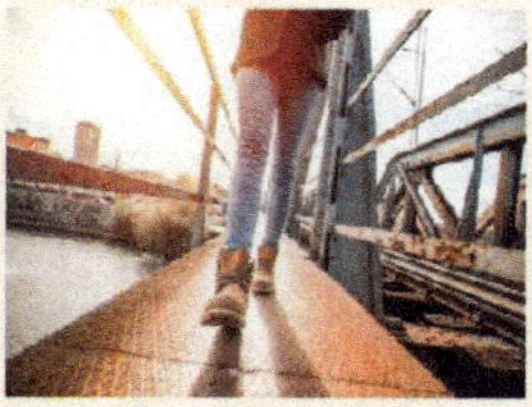

"Saying yes to happiness means learning to say no to things and people that stress you out." ~Thelma Davis

Food Allergies
Symptom Diaries

Weekly FOOD DIARY

YEAR					
___________					
JAN	FEB	MAR	APR	MAY	JUN
JUL	AUG	SEP	OCT	NOV	DEC

DATE	MEALS	SYMPTOM NOTES
MONDAY ______		
TUESDAY ______		
WEDNESDAY ______		
THURSDAY ______		
FRIDAY ______		
SATURDAY ______		
SUNDAY ______		

CALORIES INTAKE TRACKER

	Breakfast	Lunch	Dinner	Snack
SUN				
MON				
TUE				
WED				
THU				
FRI				
SAT				

Daily/Weekly Accomplishments
Reflection Time!
What went well, and What could be better

Lifestyle, Nutrition, and Fitness

Every morning you have two choices. Continue to sleep with your dreams, or wake up and chase them.

MY DAILY FITNESS PLANNER

date: ____________

GOALS

WORKOUTS

EXERCISE	TIME	REPS

WATER INTAKE

◯ ◯ ◯ ◯ ◯ ◯ ◯ ◯

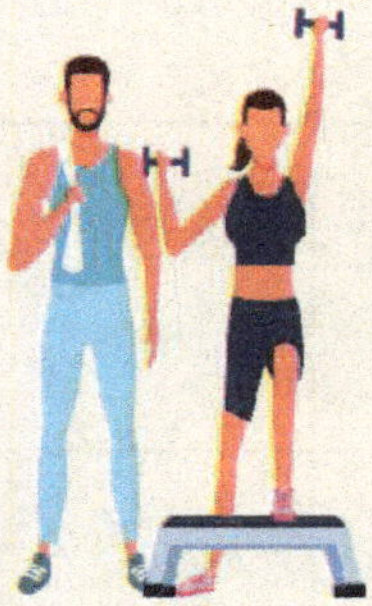

STEPS

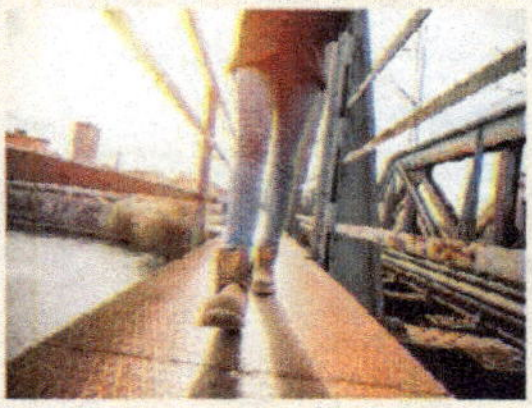

"If we could give every individual the right amount of nourishment and exercise, not too little and not too much, we would have found the safest way to health." - Hippocrates

Food Allergies
Symptom Diaries

Weekly
FOOD DIARY

YEAR					
____________					
JAN	FEB	MAR	APR	MAY	JUN
JUL	AUG	SEP	OCT	NOV	DEC

DATE	MEALS	SYMPTOM NOTES
MONDAY _______		
TUESDAY _______		
WEDNESDAY _______		
THURSDAY _______		
FRIDAY _______		
SATURDAY _______		
SUNDAY _______		

CALORIES INTAKE TRACKER

	Breakfast	Lunch	Dinner	Snack
SUN				
MON				
TUE				
WED				
THU				
FRI				
SAT				

Weekly Accomplishments
Reflection Time!
What went well, and What could be better

Lifestyle, Nutrition, and Fitness

Some people want it to happen, some wish it would happen, others make it happen. You're one of them!

MY DAILY FITNESS PLANNER

date: ____________

GOALS

____
____
____

WORKOUTS

EXERCISE	*TIME*	*REPS*

WATER INTAKE

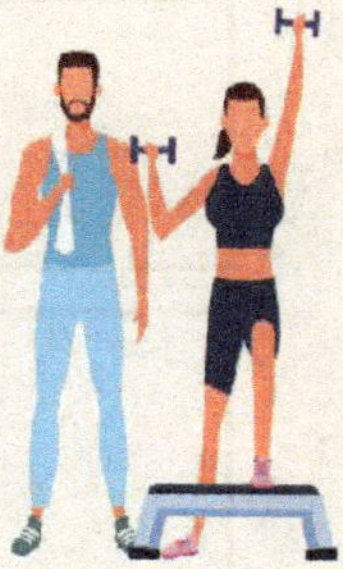

STEPS

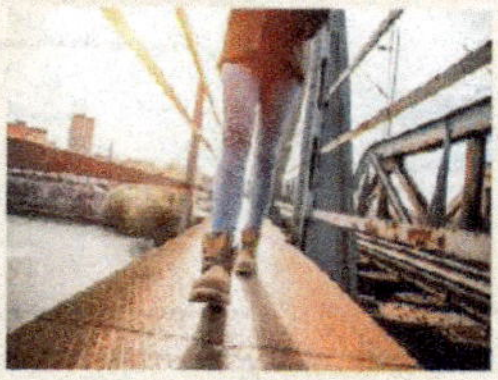

"Doing the best at this moment puts you in the best place for the next moment." – Oprah Winfrey

CALORIES INTAKE TRACKER

	Breakfast	Lunch	Dinner	Snack
SUN				
MON				
TUE				
WED				
THU				
FRI				
SAT				

Weekly Accomplishments
Reflection Time!
What went well, and What could be better

Lifestyle, Nutrition, and Fitness

Permanent results only come from permanent changes in diet and lifestyle.

Personal Reflections

Lifestyle, Nutrition, and Fitness

Congratulations! You made it here!

I'm feeling great!

Goals I've achieved so far:

What Happens When You Start to Form New Habits and Stay Consistent?

Remember when you started?

You're a totally New Person Now! Own It and Show It!

Permanent results only come from permanent changes in diet and lifestyle.

"Action is the Foundation Key to All Success" - Pablo Picasso

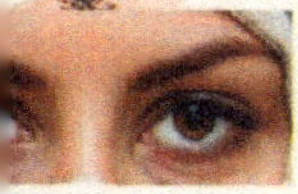

Photo Time!

Let's see Your Photo Now

Date::________

My Name is ____________________

And Today I'm feeling____________________

How You look and Feel Today

-Speak louder about your progress -

Great Job!!!

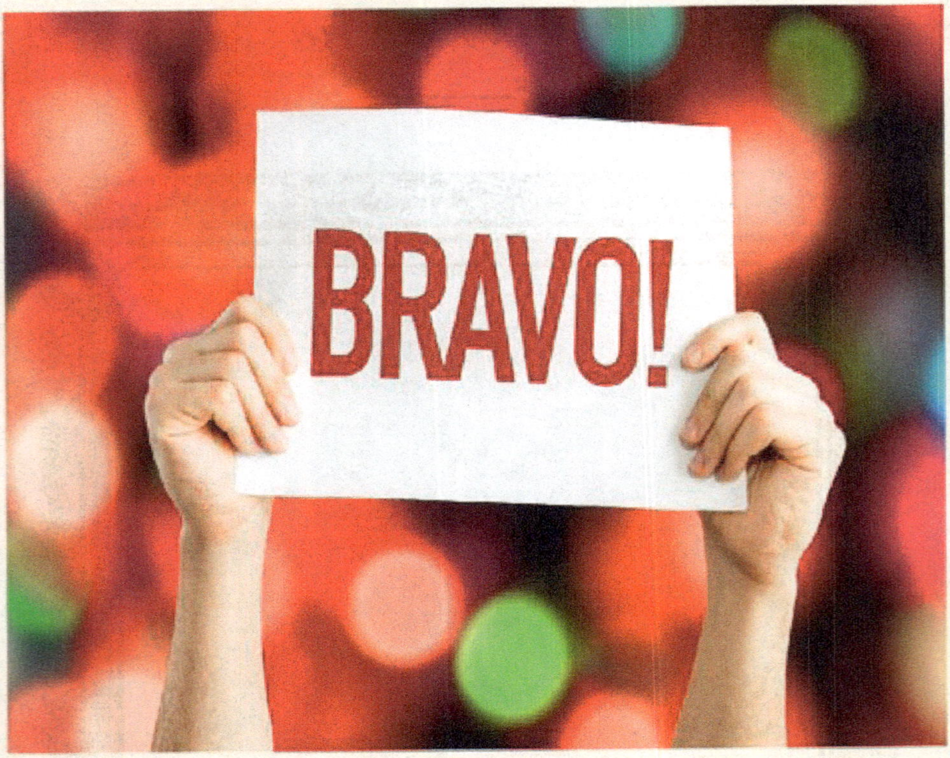

Dilcia Granville, Ph.D.

Made in the USA
Monee, IL
03 November 2026

67376432R00056